50+ Dash Diet Slow Cooker Cookbook

Enjoy the Day with This Ultimate Cooking Guide

Carmela Rojas

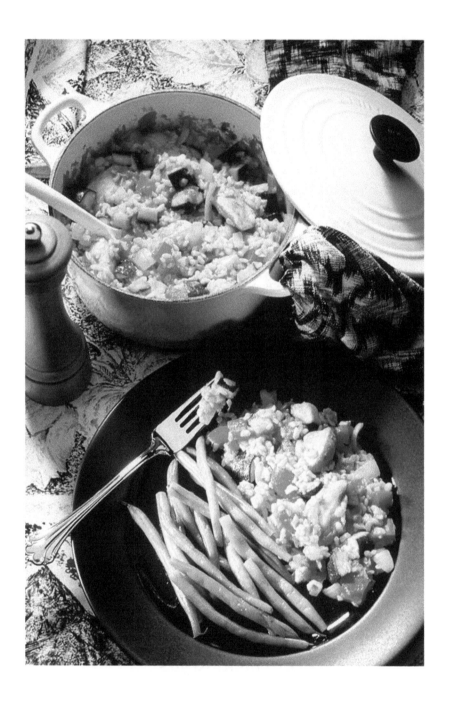

indirect, which are incurred as a result of the use of information contained within this document, including, but not limited to, — errors, omissions, or inaccuracies.

TABLE OF CONTENTS

Chicken Rice Casserole

Servings: 6 Servings

Ingredients:

- 10 ounces (280 g) low-sodium cream of mushroom soup
- 2 tablespoons (15 g) low-sodium onion soup mix
- 2¼ cups (535 ml) water
- 1 cup (185 g) uncooked long-grain rice
- 6 boneless skinless chicken breasts
- ¼ teaspoon black pepper

Directions:

1. Combine all ingredients in slow cooker. Cook on low 5 to 6 hours. Stir occasionally.

Nutrition Info:

Per serving: 187 g water; 215 calories (8% from fat, 37% from protein, 55% from carb); 19 g protein; 2 g total fat; 1 g saturated fat; 0 g monounsaturated fat; 1 g polyunsaturated fat; 29 g carb; 1 g fiber; 1 g sugar; 199 mg phosphorus; 26 mg calcium; 2 mg iron; 65 mg sodium; 395 mg potassium; 19 IU vitamin A; 5 mg ATE vitamin E; 1 mg vitamin C; 43 mg cholesterol

Orange Chicken

Servings: 6 Servings

Ingredients:

- 1½ teaspoons thyme
- 1½ teaspoons minced garlic
- 6 chicken breasts
- 1 cup (284 g) orange juice concentrate
- 2 tablespoons (28 ml) balsamic vinegar

Directions:

1. Rub thyme and garlic over chicken. Reserve any leftover thyme and garlic. Place chicken in slow cooker. Mix orange juice concentrate and vinegar together in a small bowl. Stir in reserved thyme and garlic. Spoon over chicken. Cover and cook on low 5 to 6 hours or on high 2½ to 3 hours until chicken is tender but not dry.

Nutrition Info:

Per serving: 71 g water; 164 calories (10% from fat, 44% from protein, 46% from carb); 18 g protein; 2 g total fat; 1 g saturated fat; 1 g monounsaturated fat; 0 g polyunsaturated fat; 19 g carb;

0 g fiber; 18 g sugar; 123 mg phosphorus; 29 mg calcium; 1 mg iron; 38 mg sodium; 434 mg potassium; 200 IU vitamin A; 3 mg ATE vitamin E; 66 mg vitamin C; 44 mg cholesterol

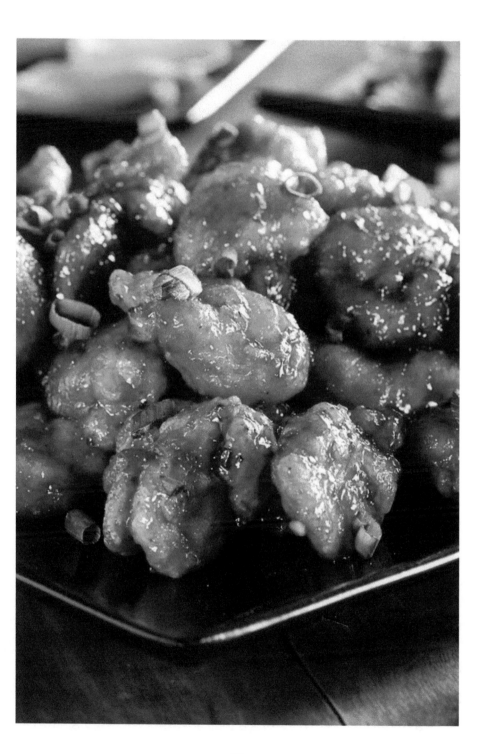

Curried Chicken

Servings: 5 Servings

Ingredients:

- 5 boneless skinless chicken breasts, cubed
- 1 cup (260 g) low-sodium salsa
- 1 cup (160 g) chopped onion
- 1 tablespoon (6.3 g) curry powder
- 1 cup (230 g) sour cream

Directions:

1. Place the chicken in the slow cooker. In a medium bowl, combine salsa, onion, and curry powder. Pour the sauce over the meat in the cooker. Cover and cook on high for 3 hours or cook on low for 5 to 6 hours. Remove chicken to serving platter and cover to keep warm. Add sour cream to slow cooker and stir into salsa until well blended. Serve over the chicken.

Nutrition Info:

Per serving: 161 g water; 173 calories (36% from fat, 44% from protein, 20% from carb); 19 g protein; 7 g total fat; 4 g saturated fat; 2 g monounsaturated fat; 1 g polyunsaturated fat; 9 g carb; 2

g fiber; 3 g sugar; 213 mg phosphorus; 84 mg calcium; 1 mg iron; 173 mg sodium; 444 mg potassium; 340 IU vitamin A; 53 mg ATE vitamin E; 5 mg vitamin C; 60 mg cholesterol

Mexican-flavored Chicken and Vegetables

Servings: 4 Servings

Ingredients:

- 4 boneless skinless chicken breasts
- 1 cup (130 g) sliced carrots
- 2 cups (340 g) frozen lima beans
- 1 can (14 ounces, or 400 g) no-salt-added diced tomatoes
- 4 ounces (115 g) diced green chilies
- 1 teaspoon cumin
- ½ teaspoon garlic powder

Directions:

1. Place chicken in slow cooker. Place carrots and lima beans on top of chicken. Combine remaining ingredients and pour over vegetables. Cover and cook on low 3 to 4 hours or until chicken and vegetables are tender but not dry or mushy.

Nutrition Info:

Per serving: 266 g water; 212 calories (6% from fat, 44% from protein, 49% from carb); 24 g protein; 2 g total fat; 0 g saturated fat; 0 g monounsaturated fat; 0 g polyunsaturated fat; 26 g carb; 8 g fiber; 5 g sugar; 277 mg phosphorus; 89 mg calcium; 4 mg iron; 221 mg sodium; 885 mg potassium; 5703 IU vitamin A; 4 mg ATE vitamin E; 27 mg vitamin C; 41 mg cholesterol

Chicken Gumbo

Servings: 6 Servings

Ingredients:

- 1 cup (160 g) chopped onion
- 1½ teaspoons minced garlic
- 1 cup (150 g) diced green bell pepper
- 1 cup (100 g) sliced okra
- 2 cups (360 g) chopped tomatoes
- 4 cups (950 ml) low-sodium chicken broth
- 1 pound (455 g) boneless skinless chicken breast, cut into 1-inch (2.5 cm) pieces
- 2 teaspoons Cajun seasoning

Directions:

1. Combine all ingredients in slow cooker. Cover and cook on low 8 to 10 hours or on high 3 to 4 hours. Serve over rice.

Nutrition Info:

Per serving: 323 g water; 122 calories (11% from fat, 64% from protein, 25% from carb); 20 g protein; 1 g total fat; 0 g saturated fat; 0 g monounsaturated fat; 0 g polyunsaturated fat; 8 g carb;

2 g fiber; 2 g sugar; 202 mg phosphorus; 41 mg calcium; 1 mg iron; 150 mg sodium; 487 mg potassium; 480 IU vitamin A; 5 mg ATE vitamin E; 39 mg vitamin C; 44 mg cholesterol

French Chicken

Servings: 4 Servings

Ingredients:

- 2½ pounds (1.1 kg) chicken pieces, skinned
- 2 cups (360 g) chopped tomatoes
- 2 tablespoons (28 ml) white wine
- 1 bay leaf
- ¼ teaspoon pepper
- ½ teaspoon minced garlic
- 1 cup (160 g) chopped onion
- ½ cup (120 ml) low-sodium chicken broth
- 1 teaspoon thyme

Directions:

1. Combine all ingredients in slow cooker. Cover and cook on low 8 to 10 hours. Remove bay leaf before serving.

Nutrition Info:

Per serving: 142 g water; 458 calories (59% from fat, 33% from protein, 7% from carb); 37 g protein; 29 g total fat; 8 g saturated fat; 12 g monounsaturated fat; 6 g polyunsaturated fat; 8 g carb;

2 g fiber; 2 g sugar; 35 mg phosphorus; 42 mg calcium; 3 mg iron; 164 mg sodium; 613 mg potassium; 1993 IU vitamin A; 0 mg ATE vitamin E; 28 mg vitamin C; 177 mg cholesterol

Curried Chicken with Tomatoes

Servings: 6 Servings

Ingredients:

- 1 can (28 ounces, or 785 g) no-salt-added diced tomatoes
- 4 boneless skinless chicken breasts, cut in half
- 1 cup (160 g) coarsely chopped onion
- ½ cup (75 g) chopped green bell pepper
- ½ cup (65 g) chopped carrots
- ½ cup (50 g) chopped celery
- 2 tablespoons (12 g) curry powder
- 1 teaspoon turmeric
- ¼ teaspoon black pepper
- 1 tablespoon (13 g) sugar

Directions:

1. Combine all ingredients in slow cooker. Cover and cook on high 2 to 3 hours or on low 5 to 6 hours.

Nutrition Info:

Per serving: 213 g water; 110 calories (9% from fat, 45% from protein, 46% from carb); 13 g protein; 1 g total fat; 0 g saturated

fat; 0 g monounsaturated fat; 0 g polyunsaturated fat; 13 g carb; 3 g fiber; 7 g sugar; 142 mg phosphorus; 72 mg calcium; 3 mg iron; 65 mg sodium; 529 mg potassium; 2063 IU vitamin A; 3 mg ATE vitamin E; 26 mg vitamin C; 27 mg cholesterol

Stuffed Chicken Breast

Servings: 6 Servings

Ingredients:

- 3 boneless skinless chicken breasts
- 6 slices Swiss cheese
- ¼ teaspoon black pepper, or to taste
- 6 slices low-sodium bacon
- ¼ cup (60 ml) low-sodium chicken broth
- ½ cup (120 ml) white cooking wine

Directions:

1. Cut each breast in half lengthwise. Flatten chicken to ½-inch (3 cm) thickness. Place a slice of cheese on top of each flattened breast. Sprinkle with pepper. Roll up and wrap with strip of bacon. Secure with toothpick. Place in slow cooker. Combine broth and wine. Pour into slow cooker. Cover. Cook on high 4 hours.

Nutrition Info:

Per serving: 37 g water; 83 calories (43% from fat, 56% from protein, 1% from carb); 11 g protein; 4 g total fat; 1 g saturated

fat; 2 g monounsaturated fat; 0 g polyunsaturated fat; 0 g carb; 0 g fiber; 0 g sugar; 114 mg phosphorus; 6 mg calcium; 0 mg iron; 89 mg sodium; 140 mg potassium; 11 IU vitamin A; 3 mg ATE vitamin E; 0 mg vitamin C; 29 mg cholesterol

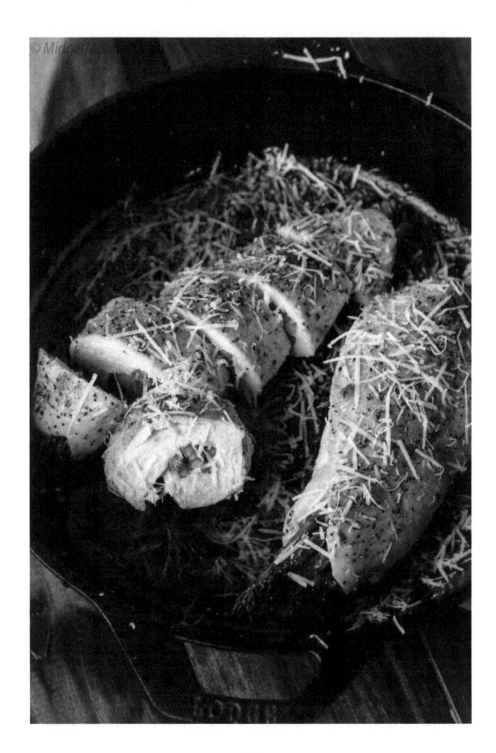

Chicken And Sun-dried Tomatoes

Servings: 8 Servings

Ingredients:

- 1 tablespoon (15 ml) olive oil
- 3 pounds (1 1/3 kg) boneless skinless chicken breasts, cut into serving-size pieces
- 1 teaspoon minced garlic
- ¼ cup (60 ml) white wine
- 1¼ cups (295 ml) low-sodium chicken broth
- 1 teaspoon basil
- ½ cup (55 g) oil-packed sun-dried tomatoes, cut into silvers

Directions:

1. Heat oil in skillet over medium-high heat. Cook several pieces of chicken at a time but make sure not to crowd the skillet so the chicken can brown evenly. Transfer chicken to slow cooker as it finishes browning. Add garlic, wine, chicken broth, and basil to skillet. Bring to a boil. Scrape up any bits from the

bottom of the pan. Pour over chicken. Scatter tomatoes over the top. Cover and cook on low 4 to 6 hours.

Nutrition Info:

Per serving: 302 g water; 288 calories (21% from fat, 75% from protein, 4% from carb); 40 g protein; 5 g total fat; 1 g saturated fat; 2 g monounsaturated fat; 1 g polyunsaturated fat; 7 g carb; 0 g fiber; 5 g sugar; 350 mg phosphorus; 27 mg calcium; 6 mg iron; 141 mg sodium; 584 mg potassium; 132 IU vitamin A; 10 mg ATE vitamin E; 9 mg vitamin C; 99 mg cholesterol

Honey Mustard Chicken

Servings: 4 Servings

Ingredients:

- 4 chicken breasts
- 2 tablespoons (28 g) unsalted butter, melted
- 2 tablespoons (40 g) honey
- 2 teaspoons prepared mustard

Directions:

1. Spray slow cooker with nonstick cooking spray and add chicken. Mix butter, honey, and mustard together in a small bowl. Pour sauce over chicken. Cover and cook on high 3 hours or on low 5 to 6 hours.

Nutrition Info:

Per serving: 42 g water; 171 calories (40% from fat, 39% from protein, 21% from carb); 17 g protein; 8 g total fat; 4 g saturated fat; 2 g monounsaturated fat; 1 g polyunsaturated fat; 9 g carb; 0 g fiber; 9 g sugar; 96 mg phosphorus; 11 mg calcium; 1 mg iron; 37 mg sodium; 119 mg potassium; 190 IU vitamin A; 51 mg ATE vitamin E; 0 mg vitamin C; 59 mg cholesterol

Asian Turkey

Servings: 6 Servings

Ingredients:

- 3 cups (420 g) cooked turkey, cut into ¾-inch (1.9 cm) pieces
- 1 cup (150 g) red bell pepper, cut into short, thin strips
- 1¼ cups (295 ml) low-sodium chicken broth , divided
- ¼ cup (60 ml) low- sodium soy sauce
- ¾ teaspoon minced garlic
- ½ teaspoon red pepper flakes
- 2 tablespoons (16 g) cornstarch
- ¼ cup (25 g) scallions, cut in ½-inch (1.3 cm) pieces
- 1/3 cup (87 g) peanut butter
- ½ cup (73 g) chopped unsalted dry roasted peanuts
- ½ cup (8 g) chopped fresh cilantro

Directions:

1. Place turkey, bell pepper, 1 cup (235 ml) broth, soy sauce, garlic, and red pepper flakes in slow cooker. Cover and cook on low 3 hours. Mix cornstarch with

remaining ¼ cup (60 ml) of broth in small bowl until smooth. Turn slow cooker to high. Stir in scallions, peanut butter, and cornstarch mixture. Cover and cook 30 minutes on high or until sauce is thickened. Serve over rice or angel hair pasta. Sprinkle with chopped nuts and cilantro.

Nutrition Info:

Per serving: 132 g water; 307 calories (48% from fat, 37% from protein, 15% from carb); 29 g protein; 17 g total fat; 3 g saturated fat; 7 g monounsaturated fat; 5 g polyunsaturated fat; 12 g carb; 3 g fiber; 3 g sugar; 277 mg phosphorus; 43 mg calcium; 2 mg iron; 141 mg sodium; 548 mg potassium; 1115 IU vitamin A; 0 mg ATE vitamin E; 34 mg vitamin C; 54 mg cholesterol

Thai Chicken

Servings: 6 Servings

Ingredients:

- 6 chicken thighs, skin removed
- ¾ cup (195 g) low-sodium salsa
- ½ cup (130 g) chunky peanut butter
- 1 tablespoon (15 ml) low-sodium soy sauce
- 2 tablespoons (28 ml) lime juice
- 1 teaspoon grated fresh ginger
- 1 tablespoon (1 g) chopped cilantro

Directions:

1. Put chicken in slow cooker. In a bowl, mix together remaining ingredients except cilantro. Cover and cook on low 8 to 9 hours or until chicken is cooked through but not dry. Skim off any fat. Remove chicken to a platter and serve topped with sauce. Sprinkle with cilantro.

Nutrition Info:

Per serving: 67 g water; 195 calories (57% from fat, 28% from protein, 15% from carb); 14 g protein; 12 g total fat; 2 g saturated

fat; 6 g monounsaturated fat; 3 g polyunsaturated fat; 7 g carb; 2 g fiber; 3 g sugar; 150 mg phosphorus; 23 mg calcium; 1 mg iron; 162 mg sodium; 363 mg potassium; 153 IU vitamin A; 8 mg ATE vitamin E; 2 mg vitamin C; 34 mg cholesterol

Chicken In Wine Sauce

Servings: 8 Servings

Ingredients:

- 2 pounds (900 g) chicken breasts
- 10 ounces (280 g) low-sodium cream of mushroom soup
- 2 tablespoons (15 g) low-sodium onion soup mix
- 1 cup (235 ml) dry white wine

Directions:

1. Put chicken in slow cooker. Combine remaining ingredients and pour over chicken. Cover and cook on low 6 to 8 hours.

Nutrition Info:

Per serving: 134 g water; 214 calories (20% from fat, 72% from protein, 8% from carb); 33 g protein; 4 g total fat; 1 g saturated fat; 1 g monounsaturated fat; 1 g polyunsaturated fat; 4 g carb; 0 g fiber; 1 g sugar; 210 mg phosphorus; 22 mg calcium; 1 mg iron; 84 mg sodium; 365 mg potassium; 24 IU vitamin A; 8 mg ATE vitamin E; 0 mg vitamin C; 88 mg cholesterol

Mexican Chicken

Servings: 5 Servings

Ingredients:

- 1 can (15 ounces, or 420 g) no-salt-added black beans, drained
- 2 cups (328 g) frozen corn
- 1 teaspoon minced garlic
- ¼ teaspoon cumin
- 1 cup (260 g) low-sodium salsa , divided
- 5 boneless skinless chicken breasts
- 8 ounces (225 g) fat-free cream cheese, cubed

Directions:

1. Combine beans, corn, garlic, cumin, and half of salsa in slow cooker. Arrange chicken breasts over top. Pour remaining salsa over top. Cover and cook on high 2 to 3 hours or on low 4 to 6 hours. Remove chicken and cut into bite-size pieces. Return to cooker. Stir in cream cheese. Cook on high until cream cheese melts.

Nutrition Info:

Per serving: 235 g water; 363 calories (24% from fat, 34% from protein, 43% from carb); 31 g protein; 10 g total fat; 5 g saturated fat; 3 g monounsaturated fat; 1 g polyunsaturated fat; 40 g carb; 10 g fiber; 4 g sugar; 379 mg phosphorus; 100 mg calcium; 4 mg iron; 305 mg sodium; 813 mg potassium; 483 IU vitamin A; 86 mg ATE vitamin E; 4 mg vitamin C; 67 mg cholesterol

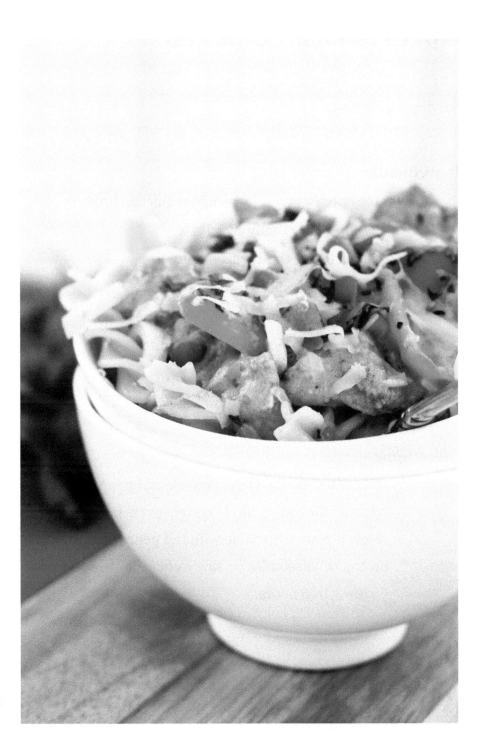

North African Chicken

Servings: 4 Servings

Ingredients:

- 1½ cups (355 ml) low-sodium chicken broth
- ½ cup (50 g) thinly sliced celery
- 1 cup (160 g) thinly sliced onions
- ½ cup (75 g) sliced red bell pepper
- ½ cup (75 g) sliced green bell pepper
- ½ cup (130 g) chunky peanut butter
- 8 chicken thighs, skinned
- ¼ teaspoon red pepper flakes

Directions:

1. Combine broth, celery, onions, and peppers in slow cooker. Spread peanut butter over both sides of chicken pieces. Sprinkle with red pepper flakes. Place on top of vegetables in slow cooker. Cover and cook on low 5 to 6 hours.

Nutrition Info:

Per serving: 233 g water; 331 calories (53% from fat, 31% from protein, 16% from carb); 25 g protein; 19 g total fat; 4 g saturated fat; 9 g monounsaturated fat; 5 g polyunsaturated fat; 13 g carb; 4 g fiber; 6 g sugar; 273 mg phosphorus; 43 mg calcium; 2 mg iron; 201 mg sodium; 621 mg potassium; 809 IU vitamin A; 16 mg ATE vitamin E; 42 mg vitamin C; 68 mg cholesterol

Italian Chicken And Bean Stew

Servings: 4 Servings

Ingredients:

- 2 boneless skinless chicken breasts, cut in 1½-inch (3.8 cm) pieces
- 19 ounces (530 g) no-salt-added cannellini beans, drained and rinsed
- 15 ounces (425 g) no-salt-added kidney beans, drained and rinsed
- 1 can (14 ounces, or 400 g) no-salt-added diced tomatoes, undrained
- 1 cup (100 g) chopped celery
- 1 cup (130 g) sliced carrots
- 1 teaspoon minced garlic
- 1 cup (235 ml) water
- ½ cup (120 ml) dry red wine
- 3 tablespoons (48 g) no-salt-added tomato paste
- 1 tablespoon (13 g) sugar
- 1¼ teaspoons Italian seasoning

Directions:

1.   Combine chicken, cannellini beans, kidney beans, tomatoes, celery, carrots, and garlic in slow cooker. Mix well. In medium bowl, thoroughly combine all remaining ingredients. Pour over chicken and vegetables and mix well. Cover and cook on low 5 to 6 hours or on high 3 hours.

Nutrition Info:

Per serving: 431 g water; 412 calories (3% from fat, 31% from protein, 65% from carb); 31 g protein; 2 g total fat; 0 g saturated fat; 0 g monounsaturated fat; 1 g polyunsaturated fat; 66 g carb; 22 g fiber; 9 g sugar; 498 mg phosphorus; 208 mg calcium; 8 mg iron; 101 mg sodium; 1544 mg potassium; 5830 IU vitamin A; 2 mg ATE vitamin E; 18 mg vitamin C; 21 mg cholesterol

Chicken Creole

Servings: 6 Servings

Ingredients:

- 2 tablespoons (28 g) unsalted butter
- ½ cup (75 g) chopped green bell pepper
- ¾ cup (120 g) chopped onions
- ½ cup (50 g) chopped celery
- 1 can (14 ounces, or 400 g) no-salt-added diced tomatoes
- ¼ teaspoon pepper
- ¼ teaspoon cayenne
- 1 cup (235 ml) water
- 2 cups (280 g) cubed cooked chicken breast
- 4 ounces (115 g) mushrooms, sliced

Directions:

1. Melt butter in slow cooker set on high. Add green pepper, onions, celery, tomatoes, pepper, cayenne, and water. Cover and cook on high, about a half hour, while preparing remaining ingredients. Add chicken and mushrooms. Cover and cook on low 2 to 3 hours.

Nutrition Info:

Per serving: 188 g water; 138 calories (37% from fat, 46% from protein, 17% from carb); 16 g protein; 6 g total fat; 3 g saturated fat; 2 g monounsaturated fat; 1 g polyunsaturated fat; 6 g carb; 2 g fiber; 3 g sugar; 147 mg phosphorus; 40 mg calcium; 1 mg iron; 54 mg sodium; 379 mg potassium; 297 IU vitamin A; 35 mg ATE vitamin E; 19 mg vitamin C; 50 mg cholesterol

Slow Cooker Roast Turkey Breast

Servings: 6 Servings

Ingredients:

- 1 turkey breast
- 2 tablespoons (15 g) low-sodium onion soup mix

Directions:

1. Rinse the turkey breast and pat dry. Cut off any excess skin but leave the skin covering the breast. Rub onion soup mix all over outside of the turkey and under the skin. Place in a slow cooker. Cover and cook on high for 1 hour and then set to low and cook for 7 hours.

Nutrition Info:

Per serving: 111 g water; 173 calories (13% from fat, 87% from protein, 0% from carb); 35 g protein; 2 g total fat; 1 g saturated fat; 0 g monounsaturated fat; 1 g polyunsaturated fat; 0 g carb; 0 g fiber; 0 g sugar; 306 mg phosphorus; 18 mg calcium; 2 mg iron; 95 mg sodium; 458 mg potassium; 0 IU vitamin A; 0 mg ATE vitamin E; 0 mg vitamin C; 90 mg cholesterol

Asian Chicken

Servings: 6 Servings

Ingredients:

- 6 boneless skinless chicken breasts, cubed
- 1 cup (130 g) diced carrots
- ¼ cup (40 g) chopped onion
- ½ cup (120 ml) low-sodium soy sauce
- ¼ cup (60 ml) rice vinegar
- ¼ cup (30 g) sesame seeds
- 1 tablespoon (5.5 g) ground ginger
- 1 teaspoon sesame oil
- 1 cup (71 g) broccoli
- 1 cup (100 g) cauliflower

Directions:

1. Combine all ingredients except broccoli and cauliflower in slow cooker. Cover and cook on low 3 to 5 hours. Stir in broccoli and cauliflower and cook 1 hour more.

Nutrition Info:

Per serving: 135 g water; 157 calories (28% from fat, 50% from protein, 22% from carb); 20 g protein; 5 g total fat; 1 g saturated fat; 2 g monounsaturated fat; 2 g polyunsaturated fat; 8 g carb; 3 g fiber; 2 g sugar; 228 mg phosphorus; 91 mg calcium; 2 mg iron; 137 mg sodium; 422 mg potassium; 3700 IU vitamin A; 4 mg ATE vitamin E; 25 mg vitamin C; 41 mg cholesterol

Curried Chicken with Sweet Potatoes

Servings: 4 Servings

Ingredients:

- 4 boneless skinless chicken breasts
- ¾ cup (120 g) chopped onion
- 2 sweet potatoes, cubed
- ¼ cup (60 ml) orange juice
- ½ teaspoon minced garlic
- ½ teaspoon pepper
- 4 teaspoons (8 g) curry powder

Directions:

1. Place chicken in slow cooker. Cover with onions and sweet potatoes. Combine orange juice, garlic, pepper, and curry powder. Pour over vegetables and chicken in slow cooker. Cover and cook on low 5 to 6 hours.

Nutrition Info:

Per serving: 155 g water; 162 calories (8% from fat, 45% from protein, 47% from carb); 18 g protein; 1 g total fat; 0 g saturated

fat; 0 g monounsaturated fat; 0 g polyunsaturated fat; 19 g carb; 3 g fiber; 6 g sugar; 182 mg phosphorus; 47 mg calcium; 2 mg iron; 69 mg sodium; 463 mg potassium; 11944 IU vitamin A; 4 mg ATE vitamin E; 19 mg vitamin C; 41 mg cholesterol

Turkey Breast With Mushrooms

Servings: 9 Servings

Ingredients:

- 3 pounds (1/3 kg) turkey breast, halved
- 1 tablespoon (14 g) unsalted butter, melted
- 2 tablespoons (2.6 g) parsley
- ¼ teaspoon oregano
- ¼ teaspoon black pepper
- ¼ cup (60 ml) dry white wine
- 8 ounces (225 g) mushrooms, sliced

Directions:

1. Place turkey in slow cooker. Brush with butter. Mix together parsley, oregano, pepper, and wine. Pour over turkey. Top with mushrooms. Cover and cook on low 7 to 8 hours.

Nutrition Info:

Per serving: 142 g water; 197 calories (18% from fat, 79% from protein, 2% from carb); 36 g protein; 4 g total fat; 2 g saturated fat; 1 g monounsaturated fat; 1 g polyunsaturated fat; 1 g carb; 0 g fiber; 0 g sugar; 332 mg phosphorus; 22 mg calcium; 2 mg

iron; 98 mg sodium; 552 mg potassium; 112 IU vitamin A; 11 mg ATE vitamin E; 2 mg vitamin C; 94 mg cholesterol

Barbecued Turkey Thighs

Servings: 6 Servings

Ingredients:

- 3 pounds (1 1/3 kg) turkey thighs, skin removed
- ¼ teaspoon black pepper
- 1/3 cup (113 g) molasses
- 1/3 cup (80 ml) cider vinegar
- ½ cup (120 g) low-sodium ketchup
- 3 tablespoons (45 ml) Worcestershire sauce
- ½ teaspoon liquid smoke 2
- tablespoons (20 g) minced onion

Directions:

1. Place turkey in slow cooker. Combine remaining ingredients and pour over turkey. Cover and cook on low for 5 to 7 hours.

Nutrition Info:

Per serving: 202 g water; 368 calories (24% from fat, 52% from protein, 25% from carb); 46 g protein; 9 g total fat; 3 g saturated fat; 2 g monounsaturated fat; 3 g polyunsaturated fat; 22 g carb; 0 g fiber; 16 g sugar; 446 mg phosphorus; 86 mg calcium; 5 mg

iron; 267 mg sodium; 1106 mg potassium; 195 IU vitamin A; 0 mg ATE vitamin E; 18 mg vitamin C; 170 mg cholesterol

Chicken And Vegetable Casserole

Servings: 4 Servings

Ingredients:

- 4 chicken breast halves, skin removed
- 1 can (14 ounces, or 400 g) no-salt-added diced tomatoes
- 10 ounces (280 g) frozen green beans
- 2 cups (475 ml) low-sodium chicken broth
- 1 cup (190 g) brown rice
- 1 cup (70 g) sliced mushrooms
- ½ cup (65 g) chopped carrots
- 1 cup (160 g) chopped onion
- ¼ teaspoon minced garlic
- ½ teaspoon poultry seasoning

Directions:

1. Combine all ingredients in slow cooker. Cover and cook on high 2 hours, and then on low 3 to 5 hours.

Nutrition Info:

Per serving: 411 g water; 211 calories (12% from fat, 39% from protein, 49% from carb); 21 g protein; 3 g total fat; 1 g saturated

fat; 1 g monounsaturated fat; 1 g polyunsaturated fat; 26 g carb; 6 g fiber; 6 g sugar; 251 mg phosphorus; 92 mg calcium; 3 mg iron; 142 mg sodium; 692 mg potassium; 3311 IU vitamin A; 3 mg ATE vitamin E; 25 mg vitamin C; 44 mg cholesterol

Barbecued Chicken Thighs

Servings: 6 Servings

Ingredients:

- 3 pounds (1/3 kg) chicken thighs, skin removed
- ½ cup (120 g) low-sodium ketchup
- ¼ cup (60 ml) water
- ½ cup (115 g) brown sugar
- 2 tablespoons (15 g) low-sodium onion soup mix

Directions:

1. Arrange chicken in slow cooker. Combine remaining ingredients and pour over chicken. Cover and cook on high 4 to 5 hours or on low 7 to 8 hours.

Nutrition Info:

Per serving: 738 g water; 358 calories (23% from fat, 51% from protein, 26% from carb); 45 g protein; 9 g total fat; 2 g saturated fat; 3 g monounsaturated fat; 2 g polyunsaturated fat; 23 g carb; 0 g fiber; 22 g sugar; 392 mg phosphorus; 58 mg calcium; 3 mg iron; 223 mg sodium; 669 mg potassium; 334 IU vitamin A; 45 mg ATE vitamin E; 3 mg vitamin C; 188 mg cholesterol

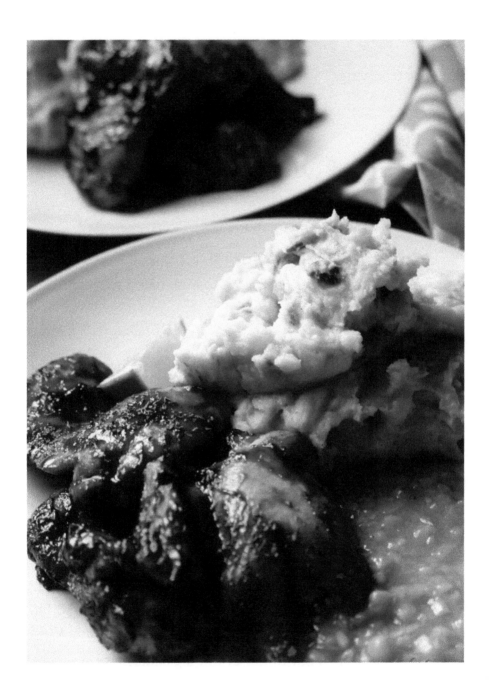

Arroz Con Pollo

Servings: 6 Servings

Ingredients:

- 1 tablespoon (15 ml) olive oil
- 3 pounds (1 1/3 kg) chicken pieces
- 1 cup (160 g) finely chopped onion
- 1 teaspoon minced garlic
- ¼ teaspoon black pepper
- 1½ cups (278 g) uncooked long-grain rice
- ¼ teaspoon saffron, or 1 teaspoon turmeric
- 2 cups (360 g) no-salt-added diced tomatoes
- 1½ cups (355 ml) low-sodium chicken broth
- ½ cup (120 ml) white wine
- ¾ cup (115 g) finely chopped green bell pepper
- 1 cup (130 g) frozen no-salt-added peas, thawed

Directions:

1. In a nonstick skillet, heat oil over medium-high heat. Add chicken, in batches, and brown lightly on all sides. Transfer to slow cooker. Reduce heat to medium. Add onions and cook, stirring, until softened. Add garlic and pepper and cook, stirring,

for 1 minute. Add rice and stir until grains are well coated with mixture. Stir in saffron, tomatoes, and chicken broth. Transfer to slow cooker and stir to combine with chicken. Cover and cook on low for 6 to 8 hours or on high for 3 to 4 hours until juices run clear when chicken is pierced with a fork. Stir in green pepper and peas; cover and cook on high for 20 minutes or until vegetables are heated through.

Nutrition Info:

Per serving: 218 g water; 599 calories (41% from fat, 25% from protein, 34% from carb); 36 g protein; 26 g total fat; 7 g saturated fat; 11 g monounsaturated fat; 5 g polyunsaturated fat; 49 g carb; 4 g fiber; 5 g sugar; 123 mg phosphorus; 75 mg calcium; 6 mg iron; 163 mg sodium; 670 mg potassium; 1933 IU vitamin A; 0 mg ATE vitamin E; 31 mg vitamin C; 141 mg cholesterol

Italian Chicken

Servings: 6 Servings

Ingredients:

- 3 pounds (1 1/3 kg) chicken, cut-up
- ¼ cup (55 g) unsalted butter, melted
- 2 tablespoons (15 g) Italian dressing mix
- 1 tablespoon (15 ml) lemon juice
- 1 tablespoon (3 g) oregano

Directions:

1. Place chicken in bottom of slow cooker. Mix melted butter, dressing mix, and lemon juice together and pour over top of chicken. Cover and cook on high for 4 to 6 hours or until chicken is tender but not dry. Baste occasionally with sauce mixture and sprinkle with oregano 1 hour before done.

Nutrition Info:

Per serving: 175 g water; 340 calories (40% from fat, 59% from protein, 1% from carb); 49 g protein; 15 g total fat; 7 g saturated fat; 4 g monounsaturated fat; 2 g polyunsaturated fat; 1 g carb; 0 g fiber; 0 g sugar; 396 mg phosphorus; 38 mg calcium; 2 mg

iron; 176 mg sodium; 533 mg potassium; 389 IU vitamin A; 100 mg ATE vitamin E; 7 mg vitamin C; 179 mg cholesterol

Mandarin Chicken

Servings: 4 Servings

Ingredients:

- 4 boneless skinless chicken breasts
- 1 cup (160 g) thinly sliced onion
- ¼ cup (71 g) orange juice concentrate
- 1 teaspoon poultry seasoning
- 9 ounces (255 g) mandarin oranges, drained

Directions:

1. Place chicken in slow cooker. Combine onion, orange juice concentrate, and poultry seasoning. Pour over chicken. Cover and cook on low 4 to 5 hours. Stir in mandarin oranges.

Nutrition Info:

Per serving: 156 g water; 147 calories (6% from fat, 48% from protein, 46% from carb); 18 g protein; 1 g total fat; 0 g saturated fat; 0 g monounsaturated fat; 0 g polyunsaturated fat; 17 g carb; 1 g fiber; 14 g sugar; 168 mg phosphorus; 33 mg calcium; 1 mg iron; 52 mg sodium; 446 mg potassium; 636 IU vitamin A; 4 mg ATE vitamin E; 50 mg vitamin C; 41 mg cholesterol

Polynesian Chicken

Servings: 6 Servings

Ingredients:

- 6 boneless chicken breasts
- 2 tablespoons (28 ml) oil
- 2 cups (475 ml) low-sodium chicken broth
- 20 ounces (560 g) pineapple chunks
- ¼ cup (60 ml) cider vinegar
- 2 tablespoons (30 g) brown sugar
- 2 teaspoons low-sodium soy sauce
- ½ teaspoon minced garlic
- 1 cup (150 g) sliced green bell peppers

Directions:

1. Heat oil in a large skillet over medium-high heat and brown chicken. Transfer chicken to slow cooker. Combine remaining ingredients and pour over chicken. Cover and cook on high 4 to 6 hours.

Nutrition Info:

Per serving: 252 g water; 177 calories (29% from fat, 40% from protein, 31% from carb); 18 g protein; 6 g total fat; 1 g saturated fat; 1 g monounsaturated fat; 3 g polyunsaturated fat; 14 g carb; 1 g fiber; 12 g sugar; 161 mg phosphorus; 33 mg calcium; 1 mg iron; 102 mg sodium; 396 mg potassium; 143 IU vitamin A; 4 mg ATE vitamin E; 28 mg vitamin C; 41 mg cholesterol

Nutmeg Corn

Servings: 6

Cooking Time: 2 Hours

Ingredients:

- 3 cups corn
- 1 cup low-sodium veggie stock
- ½ teaspoon cayenne pepper
- ½ teaspoon turmeric powder
- ½ teaspoon nutmeg, ground
- ¼ cup coconut cream
- Black pepper to the taste
- 1 tablespoon dill, chopped

Directions:

1. In your slow cooker, combine the corn with the stock, cayenne and the other ingredients, put the lid on and cook on High for 2 hours.
2. Divide the mix between plates and serve as a side dish.

Nutrition Info:

Calories 117, Fat 4.4g, Cholesterol 0mg, Sodium 266mg, Carbohydrate 19.1g, Fiber 2.6 g, Sugars 4.6g, Protein 3g, Potassium 260mg

Radicchio Mix

Servings: 8

Cooking Time: 6 Hours

Ingredients:

- 38 ounces canned cannellini beans, no-salt-added, drained and rinsed
- 19 ounces canned fava beans, no-salt-added, drained and rinsed
- 1 yellow onion, chopped
- 3 tomatoes, chopped
- 2 cups spinach
- 1 cup radicchio, torn
- ¼ cup basil, chopped
- 4 garlic cloves, minced
- 1 and ½ teaspoon Italian seasoning
- 1 tablespoon olive oil

Directions:

1. In your slow cooker, mix cannellini beans with fava beans, oil, basil, onion, garlic, Italian seasoning, tomato, spinach and radicchio, toss, cover, cook on

Low for 6 hours, divide between plates and serve as a side dish.

Nutrition Info:

Calories 715, Fat 4.3g, Cholesterol 1mg, Sodium 51mg, Carbohydrate 124.2g, Fiber 51.5g, Sugars 8.8g, Protein 50.3g, Potassium 2803mg

Stewed Tomatoes

Servings: 6 Servings

Ingredients:

- 4 large tomatoes
- 1 cup (160 g) chopped onion
- ¾ cup (75 g) chopped celery
- ½ cup (75 g) chopped green bell pepper
- 3 tablespoons (39 g) sugar
- 1 bay leaf
- 1/8 teaspoon black pepper

Directions:

1. Core tomatoes; place in boiling water for about 15 to 20 seconds and then plunge into ice water to cool quickly; peel. Cut tomatoes in wedges. In slow cooker, combine tomatoes and remaining ingredients. Cover and cook on low 8 to 9 hours. Remove bay leaf. Serve as a side dish or freeze in portions for soups or other recipes.

Nutrition Info:

Per serving: 141 g water; 61 calories (5% from fat, 8% from protein, 87% from carb); 1 g protein; 0 g total fat; 0 g saturated fat; 0 g monounsaturated fat; 0 g polyunsaturated fat; 14 g carb; 2 g fiber; 8 g sugar; 37 mg phosphorus; 18 mg calcium; 1 mg iron; 21 mg sodium; 315 mg potassium; 722 IU vitamin A; 0 mg ATE vitamin E; 38 mg vitamin C; 0 mg cholesterol

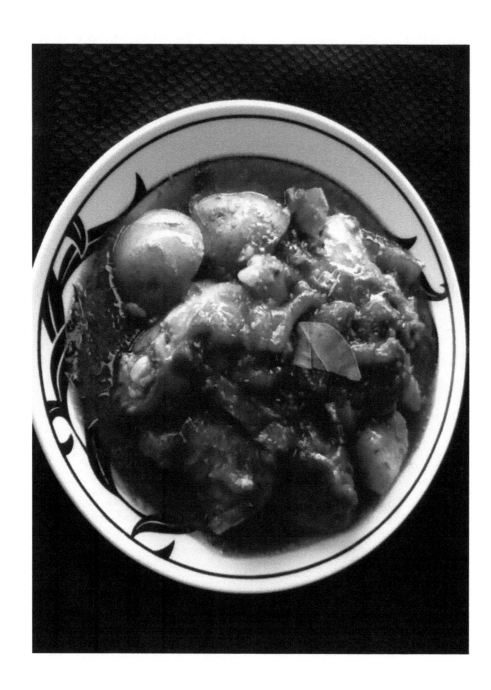

Oregano Salad

Servings: 4

Cooking Time: 3 Hours

Ingredients:

- 1 pound tomatoes, cut into wedges
- 1 tablespoon olive oil
- ½ teaspoon garlic powder
- ½ teaspoon sweet paprika
- ½ teaspoon chili powder
- ½teaspoon onion powder
- 1 cup low-sodium veggie stock
- 2 tablespoons oregano, chopped

Directions:

1. In the slow cooker, combine the tomatoes with the oil, garlic powder and the other ingredients, put the lid on and cook on Low for 3 hours.
2. Divide the mix between plates and serve as a side dish.

Nutrition Info:

Calories 65, Fat 4.1g, Cholesterol 0mg, Sodium 107mg, Carbohydrate 7.7g, Fiber 2.6g, Sugars 3.6g, Protein 1.4g, Potassium 325mg

Black Beans With Corn Kernels

Servings: 6

Cooking Time: 6 Hours

Ingredients:

- 16 ounces canned black beans, drained
- 4 tomatoes, chopped
- 1 cup corn kernels
- 1 small red onion, chopped
- 1 red bell pepper, chopped
- 2 garlic cloves, minced
- ½ cup parsley, chopped
- Juice of 1 lemon
- 2 tablespoons stevia

Directions:

1. In your slow cooker, mix the tomatoes with corn, black beans, garlic, parsley, lemon juice, bell pepper, onion and stevia, toss, cook on Low for 6 hours, divide between plates and serve as a side dish.

Nutrition Info:

Calories 311, Fat 1.7g, Cholesterol 0mg, Sodium 17mg, Carbohydrate 62.7g, Fiber 13.9g, Sugars 6.3g, Protein 18.5g, Potassium 1481mg

Stuffed Acorn Squash

Servings: 4 Servings

Ingredients:

- 2 acorn squash
- 2 apples, peeled and chopped
- ½ cup (115 g) brown sugar
- ½ teaspoon cinnamon
- ¼ teaspoon nutmeg
- 2 teaspoons lemon juice
- ¼ cup (55 g) unsalted butter

Directions:

1. Cut squash in half lengthwise; remove seeds. Divide chopped apple evenly among the squash halves. Sprinkle each half with one quarter of the brown sugar, cinnamon, nutmeg, and a few drops of lemon juice. Dot each with 1 tablespoon (14 g) of butter. Wrap each squash half securely in foil. Pour ¼ cup (60 ml) water into slow cooker. Stack the squash, cut side up, in cooker. Cover and cook on low for 5 hours. Unwrap; place squash on serving platter. Drain any syrup remaining in foil into small pitcher; serve with squash.

73

Nutrition Info:

Per serving: 255 g water; 326 calories (31% from fat, 2% from protein, 67% from carb); 2 g protein; 12 g total fat; 7 g saturated fat; 3 g monounsaturated fat; 1 g polyunsaturated fat; 58 g carb; 4 g fiber; 33 g sugar; 95 mg phosphorus; 105 mg calcium; 2 mg iron; 19 mg sodium; 915 mg potassium; 1172 IU vitamin A; 95 mg ATE vitamin E; 30 mg vitamin C; 31 mg cholesterol

Lima Beans Dish

Servings: 10

Cooking Time: 5 Hours

Ingredients:

- 1 green bell pepper, chopped
- 1 sweet red pepper, chopped
- 1 and ½ cups tomato sauce, salt-free
- 1 yellow onion, chopped
- ½ cup water
- 16 ounces canned kidney beans, no-salt-added, drained and rinsed
- 16 ounces canned black-eyed peas, no-salt-added, drained and rinsed
- 15 ounces corn
- 15 ounces canned lima beans, no-salt-added, drained and rinsed
- 15 ounces canned black beans, no-salt-added, drained and rinsed
- 2 celery ribs, chopped
- 2 bay leaves
- 1 teaspoon ground mustard
- 1 tablespoon cider vinegar

Directions:

1. In your slow cooker, mix the tomato sauce with the onion, celery, red pepper, green bell pepper, water, bay leaves, mustard, vinegar, kidney beans, black-eyed peas, corn, lima beans and black beans, cover and cook on Low for 5 hours.

2. Discard bay leaves, divide the whole mix between plates and serve.

Nutrition Info:

Calories 602, Fat 4.8g, Cholesterol 0mg, Sodium 255mg, Carbohydrate 117.7g, Fiber 24.6g, Sugars 13.4g, Protein 33g, Potassium 2355mg

Greek Eggplant

Servings: 8 Servings

Ingredients:

- 2 tablespoons (28 ml) olive oil
- 1 cup (160 g) chopped red onion
- ½ teaspoon crushed garlic
- 4 ounces (115 g) mushrooms, sliced
- 1 eggplant, unpeeled, cubed
- ½ cup (75 g) coarsely chopped green bell pepper
- 1 can (28 ounces, or 785 g) no-salt-added crushed tomatoes
- 2 tablespoons (3.4 g) fresh rosemary
- 2 tablespoons (8 g) chopped fresh parsley

Directions:

1. Spray slow cooker with nonstick cooking spray. Heat olive oil in a skillet over medium heat and sauté onion, garlic, and mushrooms. Pour into prepared slow cooker. Add eggplant, green pepper, tomatoes, rosemary, and parsley to cooker. Cover and cook on low 5 to 6 hours.

Nutrition Info:

Per serving: 187 g water; 75 calories (40% from fat, 10% from protein, 49% from carb); 2 g protein; 4 g total fat; 1 g saturated fat; 3 g monounsaturated fat; 0 g polyunsaturated fat; 10 g carb; 4 g fiber; 5 g sugar; 54 mg phosphorus; 45 mg calcium; 1 mg iron; 17 mg sodium; 418 mg potassium; 258 IU vitamin A; 0 mg ATE vitamin E; 21 mg vitamin C; 0 mg cholesterol

Thyme Sweet Potatoes

Servings: 10

Cooking Time: 3 Hours

Ingredients:

- 4 pounds sweet potatoes, sliced
- 3 tablespoons stevia
- 2 tablespoons olive oil
- ½ teaspoon sage, dried
- ½ cup orange juice
- ½ teaspoon thyme, dried
- A pinch of black pepper

Directions:

1. In a bowl, mix orange juice with salt, pepper, stevia, thyme, sage and oil and whisk well.
2. Add the potatoes to your slow cooker, drizzle the sage and orange mix all over, cover, cook on High for 3 hours, divide between plates and serve as a side dish.

Nutrition Info:

Calories 244, Fat 0.3g, Cholesterol 0mg, Sodium 16mg, Carbohydrate 56.4g, Fiber 7.5g, Sugars 2g, Protein 2.9g, Potassium 1506mg

Barley Vegetable Soup

Servings: 6 Servings

Ingredients:

- 1 cup (160 g) chopped onion
- ½ cup (65 g) sliced carrots
- ½ cup (50 g) sliced celery
- 8 ounces (225 g) mushrooms, sliced
- 2 cups (512 g) kidney beans, cooked or canned without salt
- 14 ounces (390 g) no-salt-added stewed tomatoes
- 10 ounces (280 g) frozen corn
- ½ cup (100 g) barley, not quick-cooking
- 2 teaspoons Italian seasoning, crushed
- ½ teaspoon black pepper
- 1 teaspoon minced garlic
- 5 cups (1.2 L) low-sodium vegetable broth

Directions:

1. In a slow cooker, place onion, carrot, and celery. Add mushrooms, beans, undrained tomatoes, frozen corn, barley, Italian seasoning, pepper, and garlic. Pour broth over mushroom mixture in cooker. Cover

and cook on low for 8 to 10 hours or on high for 4 to 5 hours.

Nutrition Info:

Per serving: 410 g water; 246 calories (7% from fat, 23% from protein, 70% from carb); 15 g protein; 2 g total fat; 0 g saturated fat; 0 g monounsaturated fat; 1 g polyunsaturated fat; 45 g carb; 11 g fiber; 7 g sugar; 269 mg phosphorus; 137 mg calcium; 4 mg iron; 146 mg sodium; 876 mg potassium; 1985 IU vitamin A; 2 mg ATE vitamin E; 11 mg vitamin C; 0 mg cholesterol

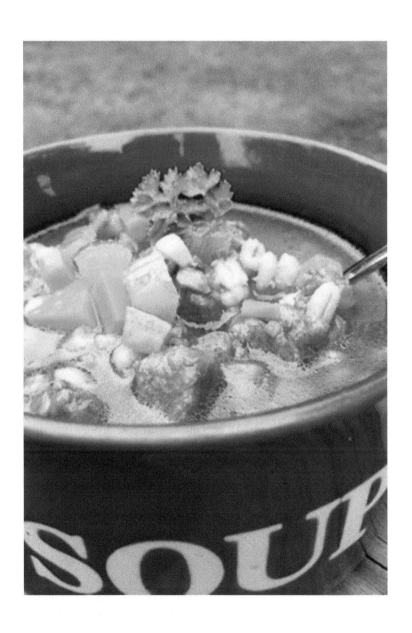

Butter Corn

Servings: 12

Cooking Time: 4 Hours

Ingredients:

- 20 ounces fat-free cream cheese
- 10 cups corn
- ½ cup low-fat butter
- ½ cup fat-free milk
- A pinch of black pepper
- 2 tablespoons green onions, chopped

Directions:

1. In your slow cooker, mix the corn with cream cheese, milk, butter, black pepper and onions, toss, cover and cook on Low for 4 hours.
2. Toss one more time, divide between plates and serve as a side dish.

Nutrition Info:

Calories 279, Fat 18g, Cholesterol 52mg, Sodium 165mg, Carbohydrate 26g, Fiber 3.5g, Sugars 4.8g, Protein 8.1g, Potassium 422mg

Orange Glazed Carrots

Servings: 5 Servings

Ingredients:

- 3 cups (390 g) thinly sliced carrots
- 2 cups (475 ml) water
- 3 tablespoons (42 g) unsalted butter
- 3 tablespoons (60 ml) orange marmalade
- 2 tablespoons (14 g) chopped pecans

Directions:

1. Combine carrots and water in slow cooker. Cover and cook on high 2 to 3 hours or until carrots are done. Drain well and then stir in remaining ingredients. Cover and cook on high 20 to 30 minutes.

Nutrition Info:

Per serving: 168 g water; 141 calories (55% from fat, 3% from protein, 42% from carb); 1 g protein; 9 g total fat; 5 g saturated fat; 3 g monounsaturated fat; 1 g polyunsaturated fat; 16 g carb; 2 g fiber; 11 g sugar; 37 mg phosphorus; 37 mg calcium; 0 mg iron; 63 mg sodium; 264 mg potassium; 13133 IU vitamin A; 57 mg ATE vitamin E; 5 mg vitamin C; 18 mg cholesterol

Cinnamon Acorn Squash

Servings: 4

Cooking Time: 7 Hours

Ingredients:

- 16 ounces canned cranberry sauce, unsweetened
- 2 acorn squash, peeled and cut into medium wedges
- ¼ teaspoon cinnamon powder
- Black pepper to the taste

Directions:

1. Put the acorn wedges in your slow cooker; add cranberry sauce, raisins, cinnamon and pepper, stir, cover, cook on Low for 7 hours, divide between plates and serve.

Nutrition Info:

Calories 155, Fat 0.5g, Cholesterol 0mg, Sodium 62mg, Carbohydrate 33.6g, Fiber 7.4g, Sugars 4.6g, Protein 1.8g, Potassium 941mg

Glazed Root Vegetables

Servings: 6 Servings

Ingredients:

- 2 parsnips, sliced
- 2 cups (260 g) sliced carrot
- 1 turnip, cut in 1-inch (2.5 cm) cubes
- 1 cup (235 ml) water
- ½ cup (100 g) sugar
- 3 tablespoons (42 g) unsalted butter

Directions:

1. Boil vegetables in water for 10 minutes. Drain, reserving ½ cup (120 ml) of the liquid. Transfer vegetables to slow cooker. Pour reserved liquid over the top. Add sugar and butter. Cover and cook on low for 3 hours.

Nutrition Info:

Per serving: 149 g water; 180 calories (29% from fat, 3% from protein, 68% from carb); 1 g protein; 6 g total fat; 4 g saturated fat; 2 g monounsaturated fat; 0 g polyunsaturated fat; 32 g carb; 4 g fiber; 23 g sugar; 62 mg phosphorus; 46 mg calcium; 1 mg

iron; 183 mg sodium; 393 mg potassium; 7350 IU vitamin A; 48 mg ATE vitamin E; 16 mg vitamin C; 15 mg cholesterol

Stir Fried Steak, Shiitake And Asparagus

Servings: 3

Cooking Time: 2 Hrs 10 Mins

Ingredients:

- 1 tbsp. Sherry (dry)
- 1 tbsp. Vinegar (rice)
- ½ tbsp. Soy Sauce (low sodium)
- ½ tbsp. Cornstarch
- 2 tsp. Canola Oil
- ¼ tsp. Black Pepper (ground)
- 1 minced clove Garlic
- ½ lb. sliced Sirloin Steak
- 3 oz. Shiitake Mushrooms
- ½ tbsp. minced Ginger
- 6 oz. sliced Asparagus
- 3 oz. Peas (sugar snap)
- 2 sliced scallions
- ¼ cup Water

Directions:

1. Combine cornstarch, soy sauce, sherry vinegar, broth and pepper.
2. Place the steaks in 1 tsp hot oil in slow cooker for 2 mins.
3. Transfer the steaks to a plate.
4. Sauté ginger & garlic in the remaining oil.
5. Add in the mushrooms, peas and asparagus.
6. Add water and cook on "low" for 1 hr.
7. Add the scallions and cook again for 30 mins on low.
8. Change the heat to "high" and add the vinegar.
9. When the sauce has thickened, transfer the steaks to the slow cooker.
10. Stir well and serve immediately.

Nutrition Info:

(Estimated Amount Per Serving): 182 Calories; 7 g Total Fats; 45 mg Cholesterol; 157 mg Sodium; 10 mg Carbohydrates; 3 g Dietary Fiber; 20 g Protein

Julienned Carrot Mix

Servings: 6

Cooking Time: 2 Hours

Ingredients:

- 1 pound green cabbage, chopped
- 3 green onion stalks, chopped
- 3 carrots, julienned
- 1 cup radish, sliced
- 3 tablespoons chili flakes
- 1 tablespoon olive oil
- ¼ cup low sodium veggie stock
- ½ inch ginger, grated
- A pinch of black pepper

Directions:

1. In your slow cooker, mix cabbage with pepper, carrots, stock, radish, green onions, chili flakes, oil and ginger, toss, cover, cook on High for 2 hours, divide between plates and serve as a side dish.

Nutrition Info:

Calories 65, Fat 2.5g, Cholesterol 0mg, Sodium 50mg, Carbohydrate 9.1g, Fiber 3.3g, Sugars 4.6g, Protein 1.6g, Potassium 304mg

Mustard Celery Mix

Servings: 3

Cooking Time: 3 Hours

Ingredients:

- 2 celery roots, cut into medium wedges
- ¼ cup low-fat sour cream
- 1 cup low-sodium veggie stock
- 1 teaspoon mustard
- 2 teaspoons thyme, chopped
- Black pepper to the taste

Directions:

1. In your slow cooker, mix the celery with the stock, mustard, cream, black pepper and thyme, cover and cook on High for 3 hours.
2. Divide the celery between plates, drizzle some of the cooking juices on top and serve as a side dish.

Nutrition Info:

Calories 103, Fat 5g, Cholesterol 8mg, Sodium 217mg, Carbohydrate 12.7g, Fiber 2.3g, Sugars 2.6g, Protein 2.6g, Potassium 353mg

Quinoa Curry

Servings: 8

Cooking Time: 4 Hrs

Ingredients:

- 1 chopped Sweet Potato
- 2 cups Green Beans
- ½ diced Onion (white)
- 1 diced Carrot
- 15 oz Chick Peas (organic and drained)
- 28 oz. Tomatoes (diced)
- 29 oz Coconut Milk
- 2 minced cloves of Garlic
- ¼ cup Quinoa
- 1 tbs. Turmeric (ground)
- 1 tbsp. Ginger (grated)
- 1 ½ cups Water
- 1 tsp. of Chili Flakes
- 2 tsp. of Tamari Sauce

Directions:

1. Place all the ingredients in the slow cooker.
2. Add 1 cup of water.

3. Stir well.

4. Cook on "high" for 4 hrs.

5. Serve with rice

Nutrition Info:

(Estimated Amount Per Serving): 297 Calories; 18 g Total Fat; 167 mg Cholesterol; 364 mg Sodium; 9 mg Carbohydrates; 1 g Dietary Fiber; 28 g Protein

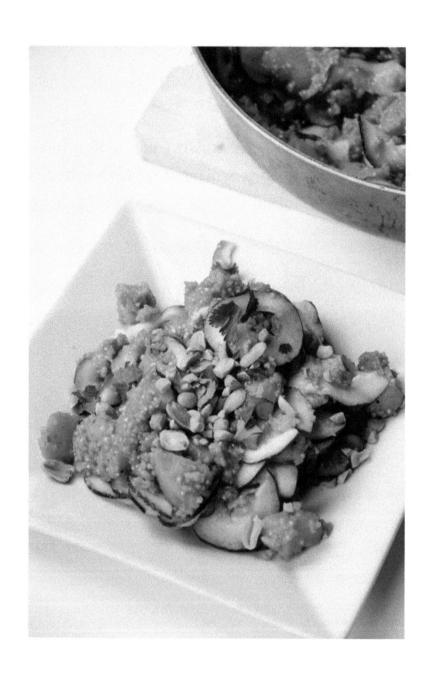

Cilantro Brussel Sprouts

Servings: 12

Cooking Time: 3 Hours

Ingredients:

- 1 cup red onion, chopped
- ¼ cup natural apple juice, unsweetened
- 2 pounds Brussels sprouts, trimmed and halved
- 3 tablespoons olive oil
- 1 tablespoon cilantro, chopped
- A pinch of black pepper

Directions:

1. In your slow cooker, mix Brussels sprouts with onion, oil, cilantro, pepper and apple juice, toss, cover and cook on Low for 3 hours.
2. Toss well, divide between plates and serve as a side dish.

Nutrition Info:

Calories 69, Fat 3.8g, Cholesterol 0mg, Sodium 20mg, Carbohydrate 8.4g, Fiber 3.1g, Sugars 2.7g, Protein 2.7g, Potassium 312mg

Italian Zucchini

Servings: 8 Servings

Ingredients:

- ½ cup (80 g) chopped onion
- ½ cup (75 g) chopped green bell pepper
- ¼ cup (55 g) unsalted butter
- 1 can (6 ounces, or 170 g) no-salt-added tomato paste
- 4 ounces (115 g) mushrooms, sliced
- 2 tablespoons (12 g) Italian seasoning
- 1 cup (235 ml) water
- 2½ pounds (1.1 kg) zucchini, cut in 3/8-inch (0.9 cm) slices
- 4 ounces (115 g) shredded mozzarella cheese

Directions:

1. In a saucepan, cook onion and green pepper in butter until tender but not brown. Transfer to a slow cooker. Stir in tomato paste, mushrooms, Italian seasoning, and water. Add zucchini, stirring gently to coat. Cover and cook on low for 8 hours. To serve, spoon into dishes; sprinkle with mozzarella.

Nutrition Info:

Per serving: 189 g water; 145 calories (54% from fat, 17% from protein, 29% from carb); 7 g protein; 9 g total fat; 6 g saturated fat; 2 g monounsaturated fat; 1 g polyunsaturated fat; 11 g carb; 3 g fiber; 6 g sugar; 142 mg phosphorus; 118 mg calcium; 2 mg iron; 126 mg sodium; 688 mg potassium; 967 IU vitamin A; 72 mg ATE vitamin E; 38 mg vitamin C; 26 mg cholesterol

Cilantro Parsnip Chunks

Servings: 10

Cooking Time: 4 Hours

Ingredients:

- 3 pounds parsnips, cut into medium chunks
- 1 cup low-sodium veggie stock
- 2 tablespoons lemon peel, grated
- 3 tablespoons olive oil
- ¼ cup cilantro, chopped
- A pinch of black pepper

Directions:

1. In your slow cooker, mix parsnips with lemon peel, stock, pepper, oil and cilantro, cover, cook on High for 4 hours, divide between plates and serve as a side dish.

Nutrition Info:

Calories 140, Fat 4.6g, Cholesterol 0mg, Sodium 21mg, Carbohydrate 24.9g, Fiber 6.8g, Sugars 6.6g, Protein 1.9g, Potassium 516mg

Corn Casserole

Servings: 6 Servings

Ingredients:

- 20 ounces (560 g) frozen corn
- 8 ounces (225 g) fat-free cream cheese
- 4 ounces (115 g) chopped green chilies
- ¼ cup (55 g) unsalted butter

Directions:

1. Combine all ingredients in slow cooker and cook until cheese and butter are melted and mixture is smooth, about 2 hours.

Nutrition Info:

Per serving: 115 g water; 240 calories (55% from fat, 11% from protein, 34% from carb); 7 g protein; 15 g total fat; 9 g saturated fat; 4 g monounsaturated fat; 1 g polyunsaturated fat; 22 g carb; 3 g fiber; 4 g sugar; 145 mg phosphorus; 48 mg calcium; 1 mg iron; 148 mg sodium; 356 mg potassium; 826 IU vitamin A; 132 mg ATE vitamin E; 19 mg vitamin C; 42 mg cholesterol

4-WEEK MEAL PLAN

Week 1

Monday
Breakfast: Tofu Frittata
Lunch: Pork Chops In Beer
Dinner: Stewed Tomatoes

Tuesday
Breakfast: Tapioca
Lunch: Creamy Beef Burgundy
Dinner: Oregano Salad

Wednesday
Breakfast: Fruit Oats
Lunch: Smothered Steak
Dinner: Black Beans With Corn Kernels

Thursday
Breakfast: Grapefruit Mix
Lunch: Pork For Sandwiches
Dinner: Stuffed Acorn Squash

Friday
Breakfast: Berry Yogurt
Lunch: Cranberry Pork Roast

Dinner: Greek Eggplant

Saturday
Breakfast: Soft Pudding
Lunch: Pan-asian Pot Roast
Dinner: Thyme Sweet Potatoes

Sunday
Breakfast: Black Beans Salad
Lunch: Short Ribs
Dinner: Barley Vegetable Soup

Week 2

Monday
Breakfast: Carrot Pudding
Lunch: French Dip
Dinner: Butter Corn

Tuesday
Breakfast: Apple Cake
Lunch: Italian Roast With Vegetables
Dinner: Orange Glazed Carrots

Wednesday
Breakfast: Almond Milk Barley Cereals
Lunch: Honey Mustard Ribs
Dinner: Cinnamon Acorn Squash

Thursday

Breakfast: Cashews Cake

Lunch: Pizza Casserole

Dinner: Glazed Root Vegetables

Friday

Breakfast: Artichoke Frittata

Lunch: Hawaiian Pork Roast

Dinner: Stir Fried Steak, Shiitake And Asparagus

Saturday

Breakfast: Mexican Eggs

Lunch: Apple Cranberry Pork Roast

Dinner: Cilantro Brussel Sprouts

Sunday

Breakfast: Stewed Peach

Lunch: Swiss Steak

Dinner: Italian Zucchini

Week 3

Monday

Breakfast: Lamb Cassoule t

Lunch: Glazed Pork Roast

Dinner: Cilantro Parsnip Chunks

Tuesday

Breakfast: Fruited Tapioca

Lunch: Swiss Steak In Wine Sauce

Dinner: Corn Casserole

Wednesday

Breakfast: Baby Spinach Shrimp Salad

Lunch: Italian Pork Chops

Dinner: Pilaf With Bella Mushrooms

Thursday

Breakfast: Coconut And Fruit Cake

Lunch: Italian Pot Roast

Dinner: Italian Style Yellow Squash

Friday

Breakfast: Apple And Squash Bowls

Lunch: Beef With Horseradish Sauce

Dinner: Stevia Peas With Marjoram

Saturday

Breakfast: Slow Cooker Chocolate Cake

Lunch: Oriental Pot Roast

Dinner: Broccoli Rice Casserole

Sunday

Breakfast: Fish Omelet

Lunch: Barbecued Ribs

Dinner: Italians Style Mushroom Mix

Week 4

Monday
Breakfast: Brown Cake
Lunch: Ham And Scalloped Pota toes
Dinner: Broccoli Casserole

Tuesday
Breakfast: Stevia And Walnuts Cut Oats
Lunch: Pork And Pineapple Roast

Wednesday
Breakfast: Walnut And Cinnamon Oatmeal
Lunch: Barbecued Brisket
Dinner: Dinner: Slow Cooker Lasagna

Thursday
Breakfast: Tender Rosemary Sweet Potatoes
Lunch: Barbecued Short Ribs
Dinner: Brussels Sprouts Casserole

Friday
Breakfast: Orange And Maple Syrup Quinoa
Lunch: Beer-braised Short Ribs
Dinner: Pasta And Mushrooms

Saturday
Breakfast: Vanilla And Nutmeg Oatmeal
Lunch: Lamb Stew
Dinner: Onion Cabbage

Sunday

Breakfast: Pecans Cake

Lunch: Barbecued Ham

Dinner: Cheese Broccoli

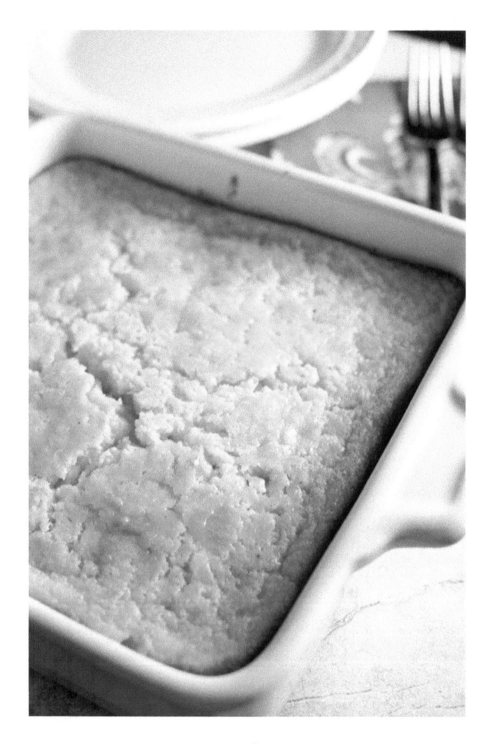

Lightning Source UK Ltd.
Milton Keynes UK
UKHW020817170621
385664UK00001B/104